I0814473

THE POCKET YIN & YANG

Published in 2025
by Gemini Books
Part of Gemini Books Group

Based in Woodbridge and London

Marine House, Tide Mill Way
Woodbridge, Suffolk IP12 1AP
United Kingdom
www.geminibooks.com

Part of the Gemini Pockets series

Text by Becky Freeth
Cover image: Shutterstock/Oksana Rybakova

ISBN 978-1-80247-281-3

A CIP catalogue record for this book is available from the British Library.

Printed in China

10 9 8 7 6 5 4 3 2 1

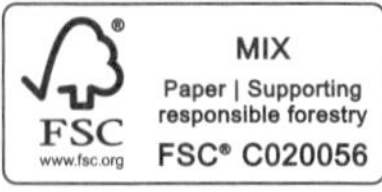

Images: Shutterstock: 3 / Oksana Rybakova; 4, 7, 15, 20, 52, 80, 108 / Elina Li; 19, 41 / Suchat tepruang; 27 / Banana Walking; 28 / Victoria Bat; 43 / Natalia Mikhaylina; 48 / Rodrigo Riquetto; 63, 64, 66 / Vips_s; 64 / Tond Van Graphcraft; 66 / About time; 78, 79 / mtedesign; backgrounds: alwaysloved afilm; Vick Lisart. Freepik / 16, 35, 36, 38, 51, 57, 68, 71, 73, 75, 85, 113, 121; 8 / kjpargeter; 116 / Raw Pixel.

THE POCKET

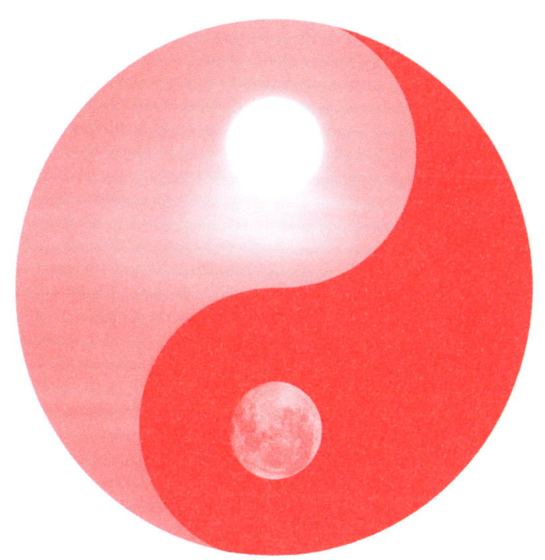

YIN & YANG

How to balance your mental and physical health

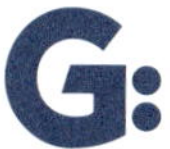

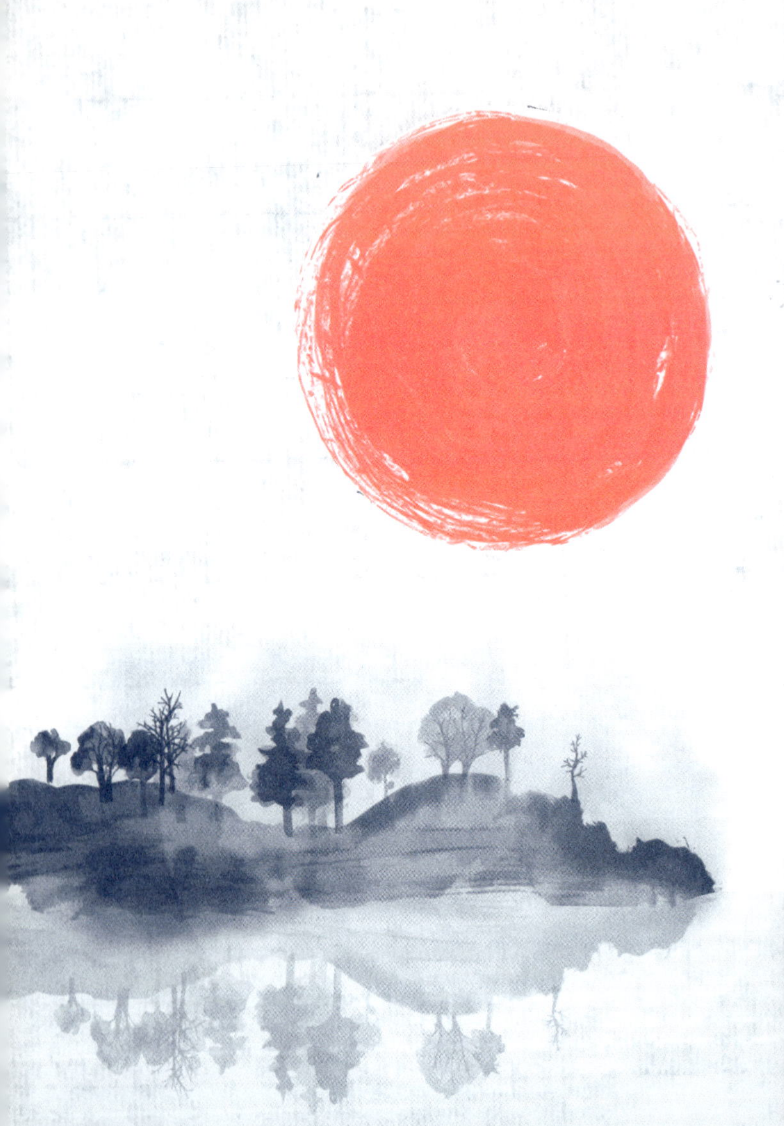

CONTENTS

Introduction

Are you seeking more balance in your life? Perhaps you want to improve your work-life management, create more harmony in the home or learn to regulate your emotions.

According to Chinese philosophy, equilibrium is the basis for a happy and ordered life because everything - from the stars in the sky to the changing seasons and even your emotions - exists on a fine balance of energy.

This is known as yin yang: the belief that all things act against an equal and opposite force. Think day (yang) and night (yin). Happy and sad.

Where are you out of sync? In this pocket-sized guide, discover how the ancient philosophy of yin yang can help you live in tune with yourself.

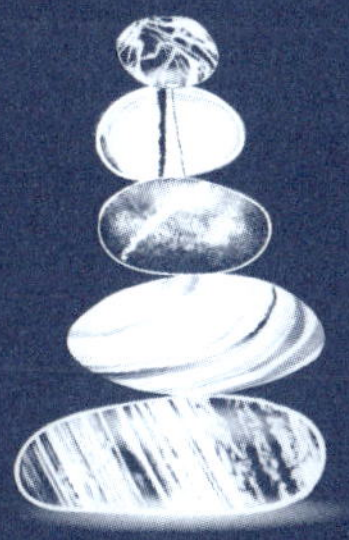

Yang energy is active and yin energy is passive; together, they create balance.

Chapter One

THE PRINCIPLES OF YIN & YANG

The only way

Think of yin yang as a way of making sense of the world: from human behaviours to natural phenomena, such as the night and day.

In the Chinese religion of Daoism, it is the only way. So where did this ancient philosophy come from and how do we apply it to our lives?

"When yin and yang were created, the lighter vapours of yang rose to form Heaven and the Sun, the heavier vapours of yin sank to form the Earth and the Moon. The yang sun creates the day, and the yin moon creates the night."

Martin Palmer,
The Jesus Sutras, 2001

Daoism

Daoists (sometimes translated as Taoists) follow "the Way" of the Universe, a path to living a fruitful and easy life.

One of the principal texts outlining this philosophy is the *Dào dé Jīng*, attributed to philosopher Lao Tzu, who offered guidance on living harmoniously during the tumultuous Warring States period (around 475–221 BCE). Though many think the ideas predate this text (possibly as early as 3000 BCE), it is one of the oldest surviving records of this Chinese philosophy, and remains a formative part of Chinese culture.

Defining all of existence

Yin yang is a core pillar of Daoism. It is the belief that interdependent dualities underlie all of creation.

Daoists believe that in the beginning, yang rose to create the fiery Sun and yin cooled and sank to create Earth. From there, all of existence could be defined by these two extremes of yin and yang.

Yin and yang are moon and sun, cold and hot, quiet and loud, and these paradoxes can be found throughout our everyday lives.

The dominance of yin or yang can change but the goal for humans is to cultivate order in all areas of life.

If yin is black, then yang is white.

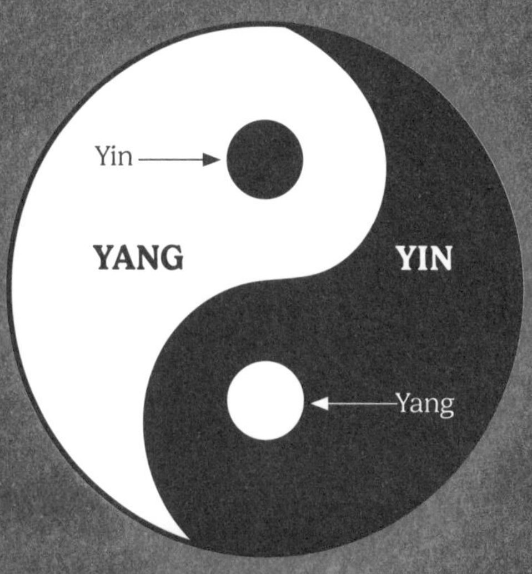
Yin
YANG
YIN
Yang

Taiji

When you think of yin yang, the Taiji (or Taijitu) symbol often comes to mind.

Now seen everywhere, from fashion to art and even homeware, the instantly recognizable black-and-white emblem has been used to signify balance since the Song dynasty (around 960–1279).

Understanding Taiji

At first glance, the two parts seem to illustrate equal opposites, where the yin half is black in stark contrast to yang in white.

But they are not static. In reality, they are ever-changing, evolving, flowing into one another. In Eastern thought, it is this interaction that powers everything in our natural world.

The Taiji may be just a symbol, but it represents many qualities of yin yang theory.

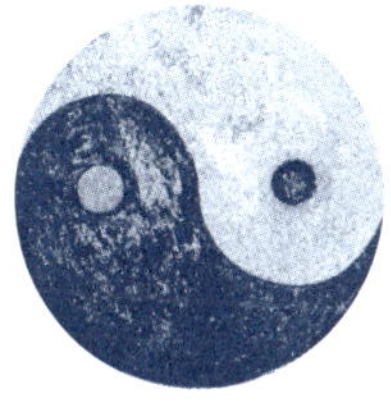

Duality

Daoists believe that everything has an equal opposite, just like the duality of black and white.

For example, yin is cold and yang is heat.

Think: wet versus dry, left versus right, round versus straight, slow versus fast, quiet versus loud.

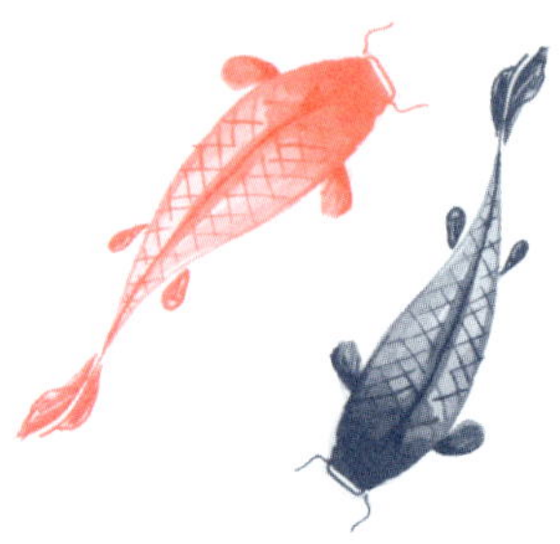

Dependence

The shapes of the Taiji are often seen as fish with "eyes" of the opposing half. The way they exist within each other shows their interdependence.

We cannot explain cold if we do not have heat to compare it to. All things are therefore relative to each other.

Dynamism

The two fluid halves appear to spiral and blend to demonstrate the transformation of yin yang and how, ultimately, one can turn into the other when it reaches its extreme.

Cold can, of course, become hot so nothing is ever completely yin or completely yang.

Wuji

If the Taiji is the interplay between yin and yang that makes up our Universe, Wuji can be interpreted as the stillness that came before it.

It is the empty circle that existed before the Universe was divided into polarities.

“Yin yang is the key.”

Robin R. Wang,
Yinyang, 2012

"The Tao gives birth to One. One gives birth to yin and yang. Yin and yang give birth to all things... The complete whole is the complete whole. So also is any part the complete whole... But forget about understanding and harmonizing and making all things one. The Universe is already a harmonious oneness; just realize it."

Lao Tzu,
Dào dé Jīng, 1992 edition

Defining all of existence

Yin and yang fail to exist without the other and are in ultimate power as a unified whole.

In perhaps the most famous passage from the *Dào dé Jīng*, it is written how one (the Dao) gives way to two (the dualities of yin yang) and two gives birth to three (sometimes interpreted as Heaven, Earth and humans). The three becomes myriad things, suggesting yin and yang are nested within all of creation.

Attributes of yin & yang

Yin yang is not a physical thing – it is more of a state – and so it can be used to classify everything we know, from the seasons to sensations we can feel. There is even yin yang within you.

It is most common to categorize things in terms of how much light falls on them.

In Chinese language, the character for yang means "sun upon the hill", so it is associated with light and day time. The character for yin means "shade upon the hill" so darkness is considered yin.

Often you will find that Chinese towns, such as Jiangyin or Shiyang, have been named according to whether they are on the sunny or shady side of a valley.

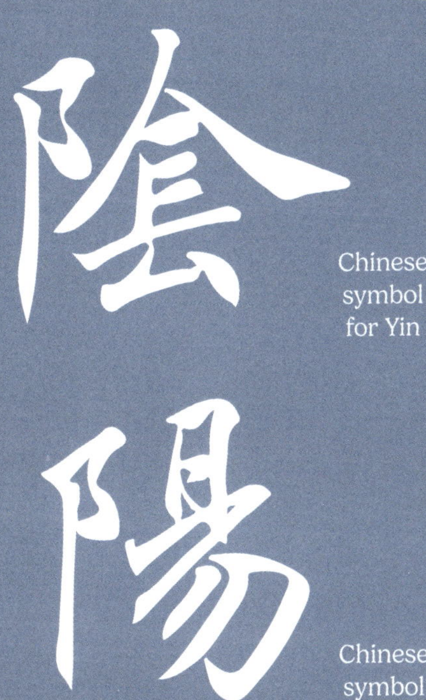

Chinese symbol for Yin

Chinese symbol for Yang

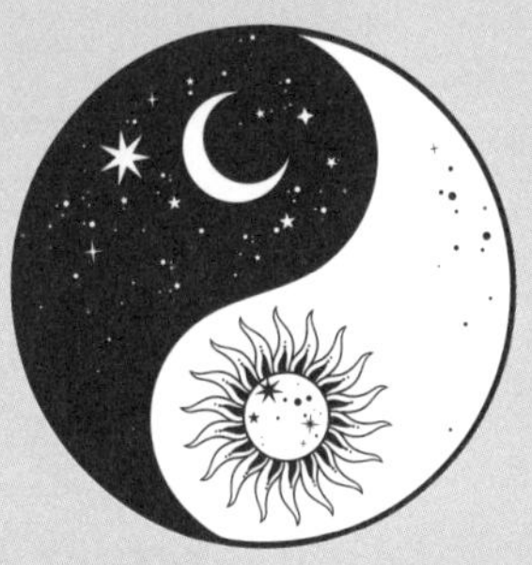

If the Sun is yang, then the Moon is yin.

It follows that yin is strongest at night time so attributes like calmness, slowness or even inactivity are yin compared to the lively movement and activity of yang.

When you consider energy and particles, you can see why yin is water and yang is fire. Yang is heat and yin is cold.

Aiming for balance

Somewhere in the middle is considered to be the sweet spot.

Think of bath water: you wouldn't want it so hot it could scald or so cold you would freeze. A soothing warmth somewhere in the middle is the perfect balance.

The same could be said of a beautiful autumn day. A happy medium between the sweltering heat of summer and perishing cold of winter is ideal no-coat weather.

Am I yin or yang?

Certain human qualities are considered more yin or more yang.

Nurturing, quiet and relaxed attributes are more yin; compared to the proactive, loud and restless characteristics of yang.

However, as the Taiji illustrates, different attributes can dominate depending on the context in which they are viewed.

Imagine a person silently listening to a speaker. The listener is yin while the speaker is yang, until they switch positions, and the first person takes their turn to speak.

There is no black & white

Remember, humans are capable of change.

A person feeling tired and introspective can boost their yang energy with exercise or social interaction.

Excess yang can cause stress that would benefit from yin activities, like meditation or introspection.

Qualities & attributes of yin

Feminine
Black
Negative change
Shade
Night
The Moon
Water
Cold
Autumn/winter
Faded
Discreet
Softness
Inactive
Stillness
Calm
Slow
Tired
Left side
Internal
Mental
Even numbers
Intuition
Quiet
Receptive
Death

Qualities & attributes of yang

- Masculine
- White
- Positive change
- Light
- Day
- The Sun
- Fire
- Heat
- Summer/spring
- Vibrant
- Obvious
- Hardness
- Active
- Movement
- Energetic
- Fast
- Lively
- Right side
- Open spaces
- Physical
- Odd numbers
- Logic
- Loud
- Giving
- Life

Transformation

Our experience of yin yang will always be somewhere on a spectrum within the two extremes.

Think of the Taiji: yin and yang always exist within the other; they are constantly moving. The transformation point of the Taiji shows that where one is at its strongest, it gives way to the other at its weakest.

Perhaps without being aware of it, we witness this transformation every day. Within a 24-hour period, we transition from day to night, and the Sun makes way for the Moon. Noon would be the strongest yang phase and midnight would be strongest yin - but, in between, there will be some yang (the black circle) in the strongest yin period (predominantly yin), and some yin (the white circle) in the strongest yang period (predominantly yang), until they reach the point of transformation.

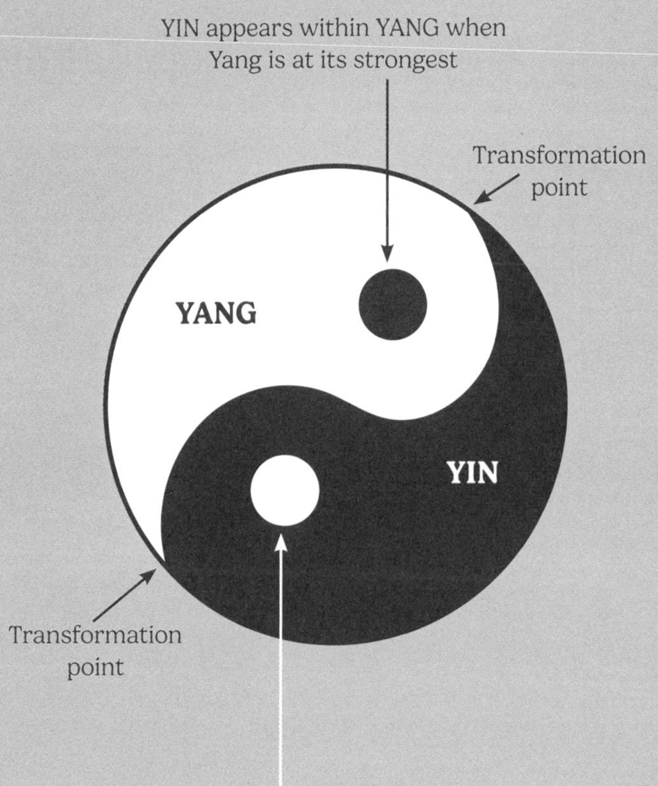
YIN appears within YANG when
Yang is at its strongest
Transformation
point
YANG
YIN
Transformation
point
YANG appears within YIN when
Yin is at its strongest

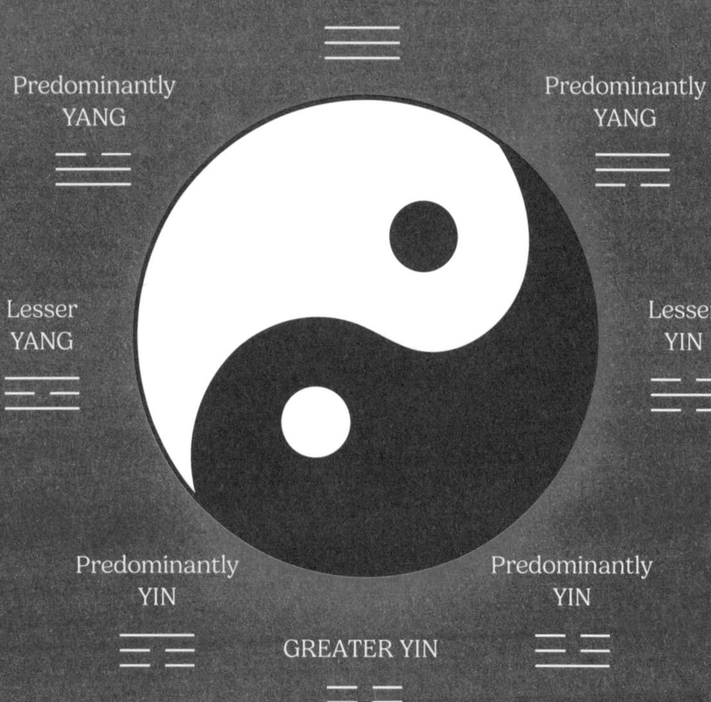
GREATER YANG
Predominantly YANG
Predominantly YANG
Lesser YANG
Lesser YIN
Predominantly YIN
Predominantly YIN
GREATER YIN

Moving between yin & yang

How do you track this constantly changing interaction between yin and yang?

As early as 3000 BCE, humans have used three-line diagrams (or trigrams) to illustrate the layers of yin yang that exist between the two polarities. At the extreme, there is "greater" yin or yang; in between there will be stages where one is dominant, while the other exists ("predominantly" yin or yang), and stages where one is at its least – "lesser" yin or yang.

Toss a coin three times and you will only ever get eight different outcomes. If yin and yang are two sides of that coin, you can visualize these variations using a combination of broken lines (representing yin) or unbroken/solid lines (representing yang) and each outcome makes a trigram that will show yin or yang in greater dominance.

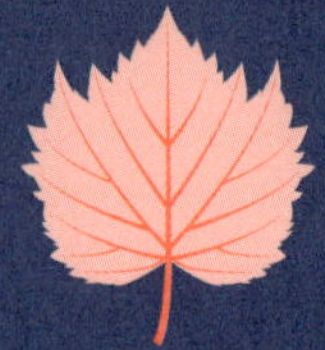

The seasons

If yin and yang are two parts of a whole, how do we categorize the four seasons?

The time of year can be determined by how much sun we experience in a day.

Spring is a lesser yang season where the Sun is returning for longer periods.

Summer is the most yang season with the longest hours of sunlight.

Autumn is a lesser yin season in between, where the hours of sunlight are diminishing.

Winter is the most yin period as it is the darkest.

The fifth season

The Chinese identify a fifth season that is often overlooked in Western society.

Instead of seeing an abrupt switch from spring to summer or summer to autumn, they observe a period of transformation between each, which is considered a fifth season.

Each transition has its own yin or yang properties depending on the quality of sunlight available.

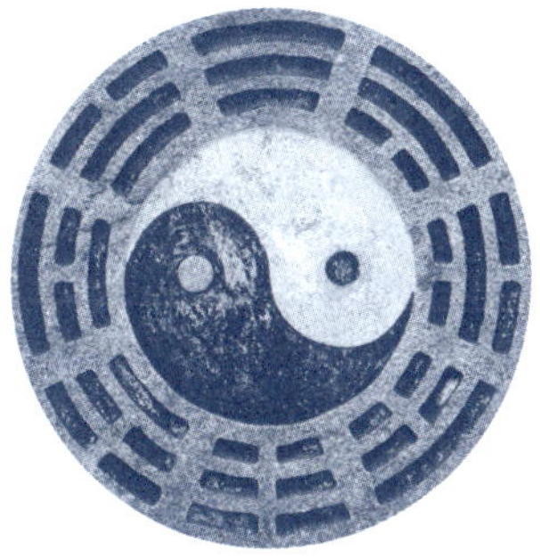

The **equinox** (when day and night are approximately of equal length) is the point of equality for yin yang, in the middle of this transformation period.

The **solstice** (marked by the longest or shortest days of the year) is when either yin or yang is at its strongest and its counterpart the weakest.

The elements

Chinese philosophy identifies five elements that make up our natural world: fire, earth, metal, water and wood.

They can each be associated with a season of the year and therefore relate to the cycle of yin and yang.

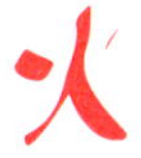

Fire is associated with summer heat and light and is therefore a yang element.

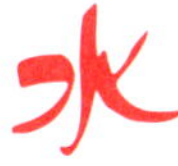

Water is linked to the cold, wet and dark yin of winter.

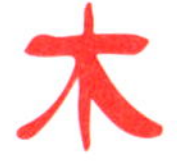

Wood is spring in lesser yin and the regeneration of plant life.

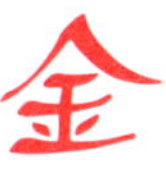

Metal is a lesser yang element associated with the autumn and tools needed to harvest.

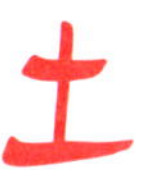

Earth is the fifth element, the source of everything, and it represents change in a similar way to the fifth season.

“We are part of the natural environment; we grow out of it in the same way that a wave emerges from the ocean or a tree grows in the forest.”

Kenneth S. Cohen,
The Way of Qigong, 1999

Wuxing

The term "wuxing" refers to how the five elements move. Each one is said to have an effect on another element, whether that is to build it up or break it down.

The most commonly used and understood forms of wuxing are the generating and controlling cycles.

Generating cycle

Each element creates and nourishes the next, such as water feeds wood in a forest and wood feeds fire.

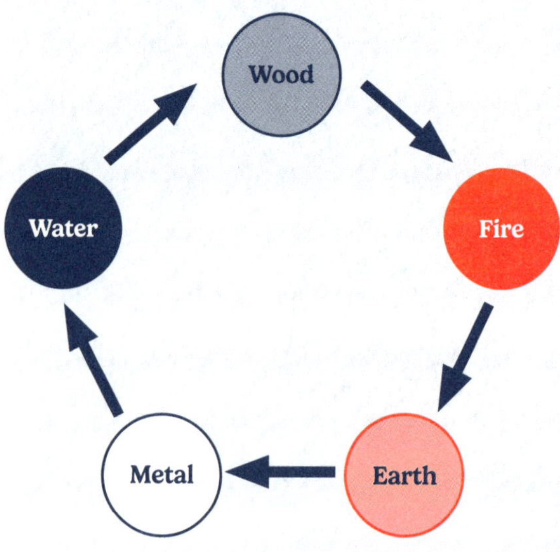

Controlling cycle

Each element has a destructive effect on another to prevent it getting out of control. For example, water regulates fire and fire shapes metal.

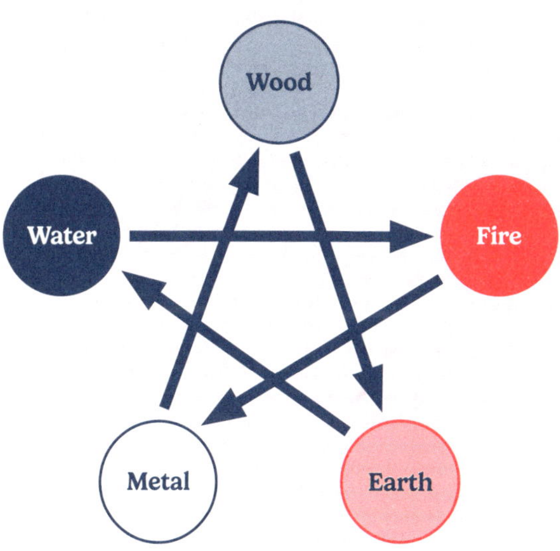

Energy (chi/qi)

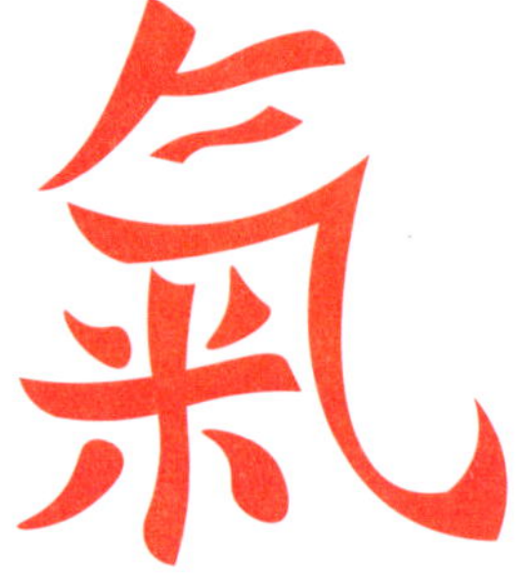

Everything in the Universe is made up of energy: from the paper on your desk and the chair you rest on, to your body's organs, tissues and brain.

In Traditional Chinese Medicine (TCM), the energy that controls our physical state is "chi" (sometimes qi).

If you visualize yin yang as the cord that connects all life together, chi is the electricity running through it. It is the life force.

In much the same way as a severed cord, anything that obstructs the flow of chi around the body is the route of all mental and physical problems, according to TCM.

The Chinese have devised many techniques to improve the flow of chi such as meditation, massage and martial arts.

Dispelling myths & misconceptions

"Yin and yang are like good and bad."
Actually, good and bad are ways of interpreting our world, not ways of explaining it.

"If you're yin, you can't be yang."
The dualities are not absolute. They are dynamic and constantly changing.

"The seasons can't be yin or yang."
Daoists compare the seasons to each other, identifying them as "more yin or yang" than the other.

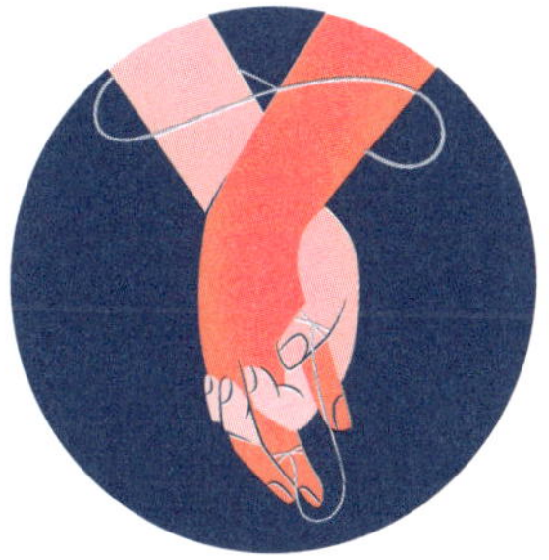

"Soulmates happen when a yin meets a yang."
People are a mix of yin and yang – and a strong, healthy bond is a balance of these energies.

"Yin is negative, so it must represent evil."
In yin yang philosophy, the terms negative and positive are used as they would to describe a magnet, in terms of their energetic charge, and not their moral value.

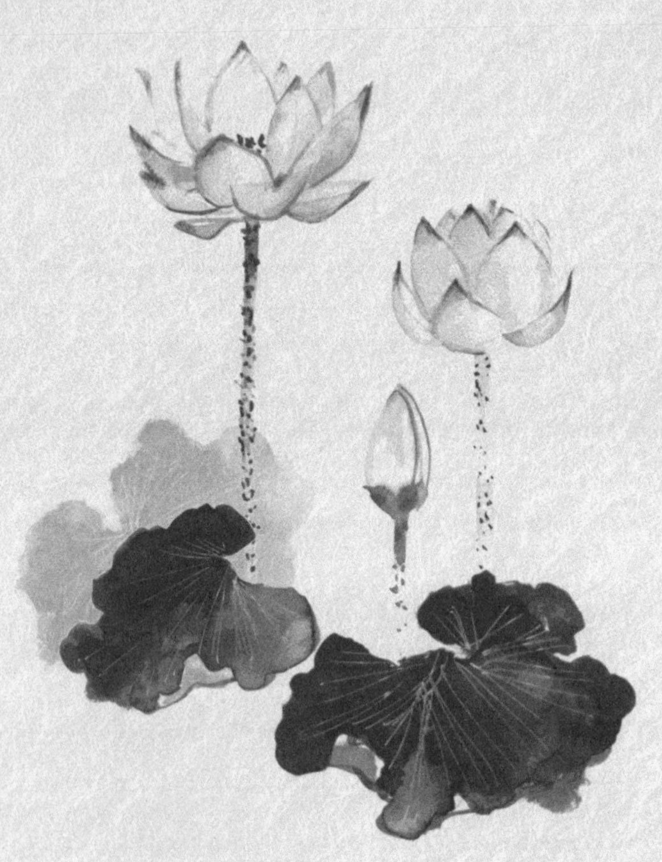

Chapter Two

BALANCE FOR HEALTH

"T'ai Chi is born from Wuji and is the mother of yin and yang. In motion, they separate, in stillness they combine."

Waysun Liao,
T'ai Chi Classics, 2000

The elixir of life

Like everything else in the Universe, you are made up of both yin and yang energy.

Whether it is pain, illness, anxiety or unhappiness that ails you, you will discover yin yang theory within countless Chinese remedies where striving for balance is seen as the elixir of life.

Movement

Exercise as part of a healthy lifestyle is not a ground-breaking suggestion, although in Chinese culture, overexerting yourself can actually do more harm than good.

If you're feeling exhausted after the gym, it could be that vigorous physical activity is depleting your powerful yang energy and leaving you feeling off-balance.

The Chinese way of movement is slower, gentler and sometimes meditative.

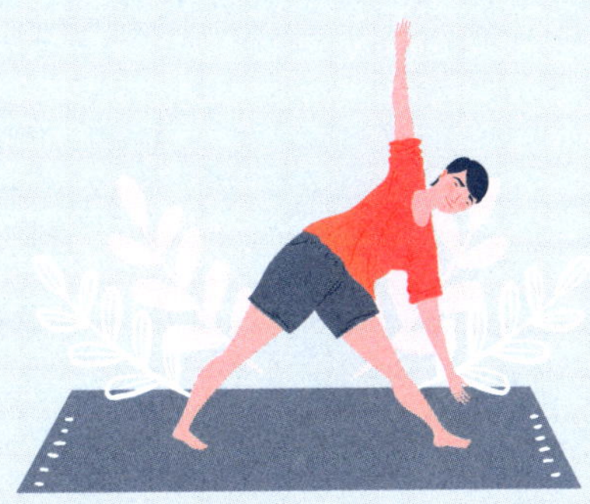

Often exercise will take place outdoors, not only because the proximity to nature is grounding, but the fresh air and oxygen are thought to enhance the flow of chi and help to detox the mind.

One of the best-known exercises derived from yin yang theory is T'ai Chi.

T'ai Chi & yin yang

T'ai Chi is a martial art focused on the interplay between stillness and movement.

It is a fundamentally yin yang practice aimed at counterbalancing soft and yielding (yin) with hard and attacking (yang).

An opponent represents the equal, opposing force and your role is to neutralize whatever is coming at you with a balancing movement.

Benefits of regular T'ai Chi include:

- ☯ Stress relief by centring the mind
- ☯ Increased blood flow
- ☯ Improved concentration
- ☯ Better balance in movement
- ☯ Greater strength and flexibility
- ☯ Increased energy and stamina
- ☯ Improved muscle tone

“T’ai Chi is about the balance of yin and yang. If you use hardness to resist force, then both sides will break. T’ai Chi meets hardness with softness, so incoming force exhausts itself.”

Clare Pooley,
The Authenticity Project, 2020

A 30-second intro to T'ai Chi

- Standing up, transfer your weight into your left leg. This has become your solid supporting leg (yang).
- Your right leg is empty (yin) and does not hold your weight.
- Transfer your weight slowly, effortlessly from your left leg into your right leg and back again.
- You are demonstrating the smooth transfer of power from yang into yin and yin into yang.

Yoga & yin yang

Yoga is a discipline of balance and alignment. So, it may be no surprise to learn that Chinese theories on energy have influenced some modern adaptations of the Indian practice of yoga.

Down to the most fundamental component of yoga – the breathwork – there is a yin element of inhalation opposing the yang of exhalation.

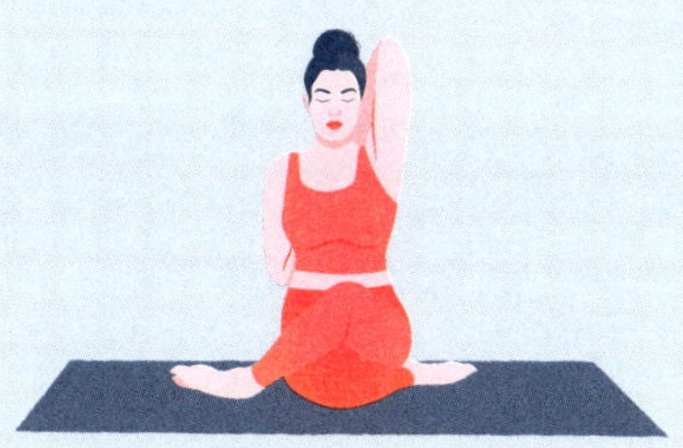

Typically, a yoga sequence comprises yin and yang sections where slow movements and stretches build into a dynamic, active flow, and eventually come back to stillness at the end.

No matter whether you come to the mat feeling too yin or too yang, you will find the harmonizing energy to clear the mind and connect deeply with the body.

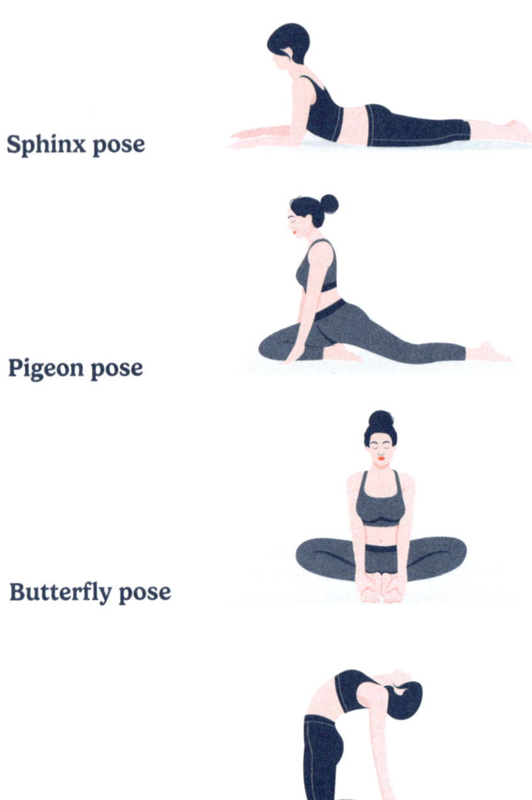
Sphinx pose
Pigeon pose
Butterfly pose
Camel pose

Yin yoga

If you practise yoga, you may be looking for peace, calm and head space. A moment of yin in a yang world.

"Yin yoga" is a slow-moving style of yoga popularized in the 1970s to help connect the physical body with the emotional body. By holding postures for longer, you go deeper into stretches, helping to open up the connective tissues and unblock stagnant energy or locked emotion.

Benefits include: stress relief, increased blood flow, decreased anxiety, greater flexibility.

Warrior 1 pose

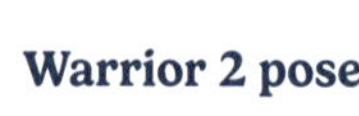

Warrior 2 pose

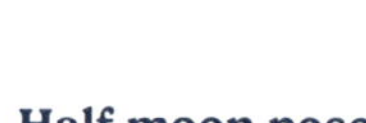

Half moon pose

Reverse half moon pose

Yang yoga

Though it's not always called "yang yoga", styles like Hatha and Ashtanga are much more weighted toward powerful poses like Warrior 1 and 2, which demand great muscle strength and help develop stamina and flexibility.

Often these active styles move faster, to a repetitive rhythm, and sometimes include a heated element to boost yang energy.

Benefits include: detoxification, increased energy, boosting the immune system.

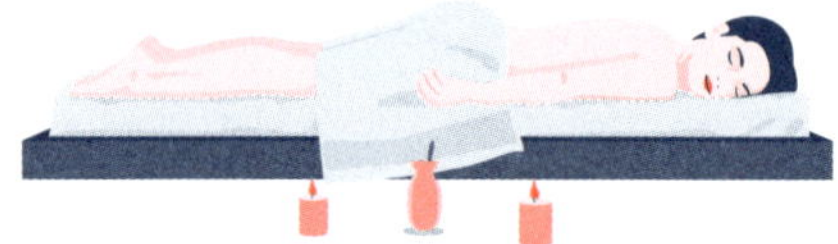

Massage

A massage is always a good idea. When it feels like parts of your body are pulling more weight than others, skilled practitioners can help to maintain a healthy level of yin and yang.

Benefits include: stress and anxiety relief, improved sleep, reduction in chronic pain.x

Shiatsu is a Japanese form of massage derived from Chinese yin yang principles where the aim is to improve the flow of chi around the body.

Sleep

In TCM, sleep is an essential part of regulating yin and yang energy. As day progresses to night, active yang is supposed to give way to restful yin, partly to indulge in the peaceful solace of night time but also to restore our energy for the following day.

This harmony of wake and sleep mimics the natural cycles of the Sun and Moon, light and dark, night and day.

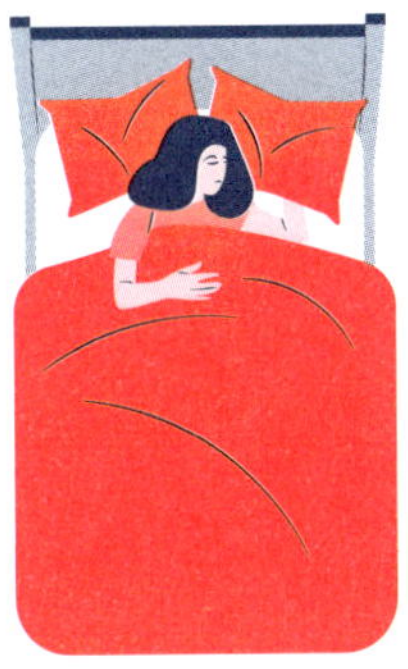

An unhealthy balance of yin yang when it comes to sleep, perhaps due to lifestyle factors like consuming caffeine (excess yang) or napping in the day (excess yin), can lead to insomnia and subsequent health problems.

5 habits for healthy sleep

1. Nourish the body with yin foods like spinach and black beans. Spices, caffeine and alcohol boost yang energy and disrupt sleep.

2. Clear the mind when you get into bed by replacing music or podcasts with meditative rituals that empty your thoughts.

3. Dim the lights early in the evening, including bright screen devices that send out powerful yang energy when you are supposed to be settling into yin.

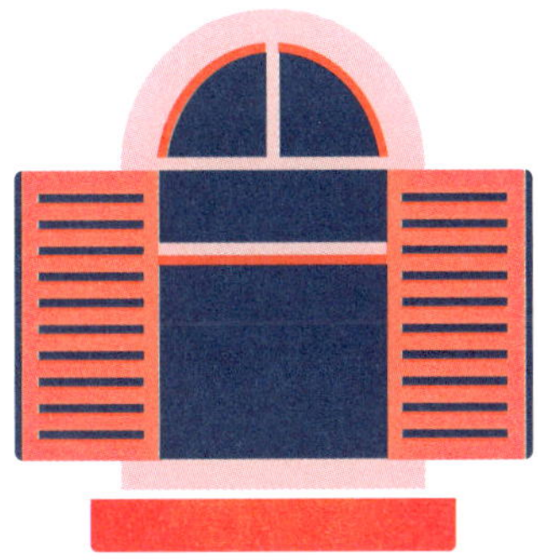

4. Open the windows to keep your sleep space cool. Waking up hot and sweaty will diminish your yin energy.

5. Wash your feet. In TCM, water has yin properties and therefore a simple and cleansing ritual can aid sleep and self-care.

Acupuncture

This ancient therapeutic technique involves the delicate placement of needles through the skin to stimulate sensory nerves, and requires a specialist practitioner.

It is a medically approved treatment most commonly used to relieve pain in athletes, cancer patients and arthritis sufferers.

It originated nearly 3,000 years ago in China and those who still apply the traditional method are aiming to correct the flow of chi around the body.

Yin yang & the body

A simple diagram of the body's energy channels.

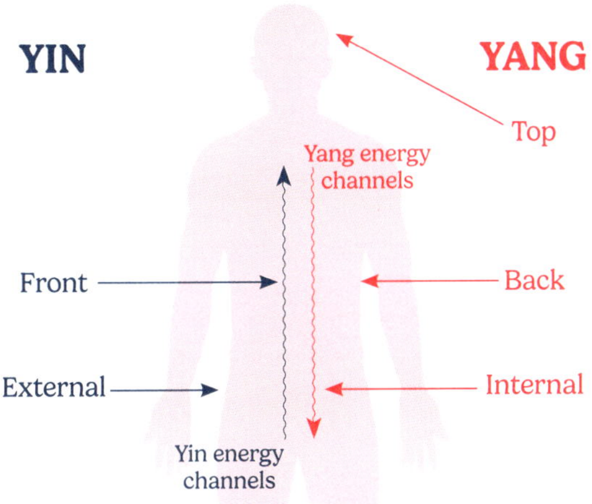

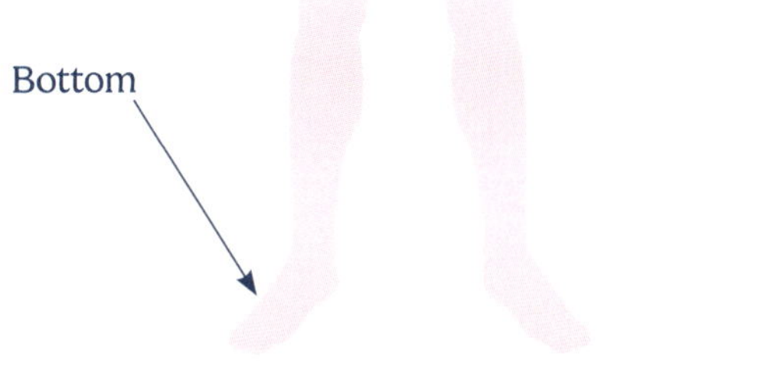

Diet

In the western world, the idea of a balanced diet is about maintaining a healthy weight with a variety of nutrients.

In yin yang theory, foods can be divided into hot, cold, warm or cool, depending on whether they fire up (yang) or water down (yin) our digestive systems.

It follows that fried foods, eggs and sweet potatoes would be yang foods because they are rich, energizing and often served hot; while cucumber, lettuce and watermelon are all yin, cooling and refreshing.

It's less intuitive that oats and peanuts have yang energy, while broccoli and tomatoes would have yin energy, as they can all be served hot or cold.

In other words, this is not about how you heat your food, but rather how your food heats you.

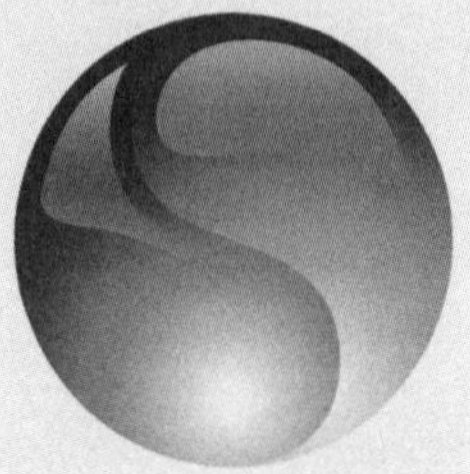

Keep your cool

Stress, anxiety and constipation are linked to a build-up of yang energy. Cold and cool foods that slow down the system and calm the mind can reduce your yang energy and increase yin.

For a yang imbalance, eat bananas, beans, spinach, yogurt and honey.

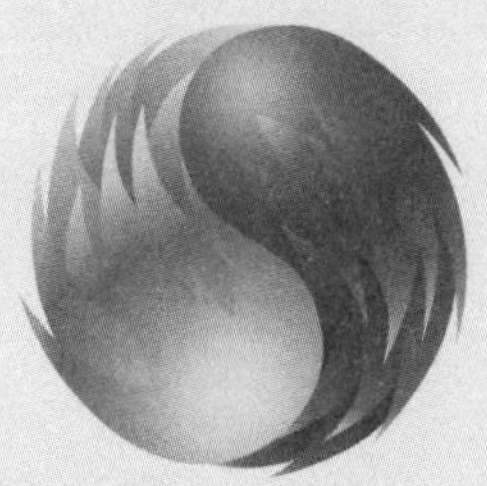

Playing with fire

Fatigue, bloating and a slow metabolism are associated with an excess of yin in the body. Warm and hot foods are said to reduce yin energy and increase yang energy by firing up the mind and body functions to provide a quick source of energy.

For a yin imbalance, eat peppers, salmon, garlic, beef and chicken.

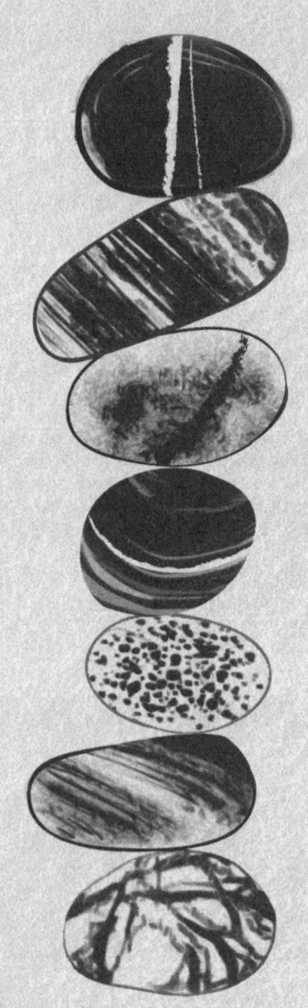

Chapter Three

BALANCE FOR EMOTIONS

"If you are hard, hard things will befall you. If you are soft, you can bend and survive. If you compete, the world will take you on. If you are able to be content, The world will roll on with you."

Martin Palmer,
Yin & Yang, 1997

Balance within yourself

The concept of yin yang is engrained in popular culture: "You are the yin to my yang," is often said in friendships and love stories when opposites attract.

But can your emotions ever be "too yin" or "too yang"?

Finding balance is believed to be the key to your relationship with yourself and others.

Male vs female energy

Traditionally, yin (with its soft, passive and receptive properties) is associated with feminine energy, while yang (which is active and fiery) is masculine.

It's important to note that this is not necessarily about gender. Any person (however they identify) can be more yin or more yang, depending on their energy.

If you think back to the Taiji, each side features part of the other, which suggests that you have both forces within you.

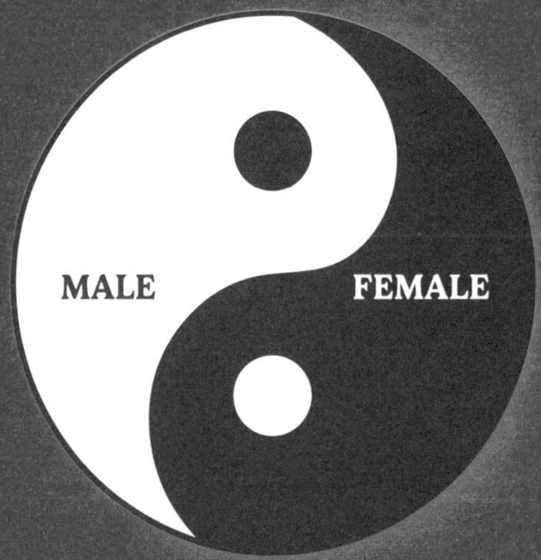

It is important to maintain a healthy balance of both male and female energies, as each can come into dominance whenever the right situation arises.

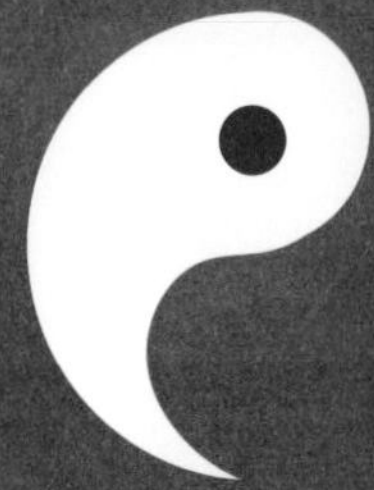

Yang characteristics

Loud

Extroverted

Sometimes fiery

Often leads a busy, active lifestyle

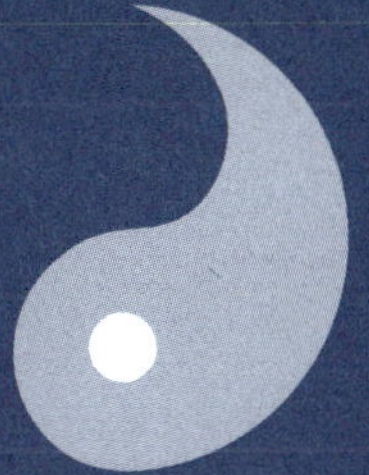

Yin characteristics

Quiet

Introverted

Receptive

Nurturing

Empathetic

Fosters strong emotional connections over superficial ones

Responding to your emotions & energy

Ask yourself, are you feeling creative, active, high on energy or a bit frantic? This could mean that passive yin activities like massage, sleep and deep contemplation will level you out.

Alternatively, if you are sad, still, bored or avoidant, you could benefit from yang physical activity and new challenges.

“There are no greater adversaries than yin and yang, because nothing in Heaven or on Earth escapes them. But it is not yin and yang that do this, it is your heart that makes it so.”

Zhuangzi
(4th century BCE)

Live in tune with yourself

By paying attention to your emotions you will be able to make healthy choices that benefit your behaviour and lifestyle.

Not only can this perspective help you to live in harmony with yourself, it can also aid you when addressing conflict.

By accepting that qualities you don't appreciate in others are also dormant within you, it is possible to find a way to relate to people who you may not initially understand or agree with.

Yin yang & relationships

Recent thought leaders, such as Professor Robin R. Wang, have broken down the interplay between the yin and yang of relationships in six ways:

1 Conflict

2 Interdependence

3 Power

4 Change

5 Support

6 Flow

Handling conflict

By the very nature of opposites, there is a suggestion of conflict. In relationships, finding harmony in this duality is sometimes about changing your position, as both of you move to find middle ground or accept a different point of view.

If one or other of you refuses to see things from another perspective, your energy acts as an unstoppable force coming at an immovable object.

Interdependence

In relationships, you are constantly moving and shaping each other.

In the Taiji symbol, yin only appears when yang is at its strongest (and vice versa), suggesting that the opposing force will always make way for the other in a cyclical, flowing fashion.

Welcome change in your relationship, just as the Taiji moves to welcome in the new force at the end of each peak.

Power

Just as yin and yang exist within the eye of each other, the balance of power within relationships can swing from one person to the other.

Sometimes yang energy is what is needed and sometimes it is yin.

A successful relationship relies on this balance of power ebbing and flowing, and not on one partner being a dominant force. Yin yang requires flow, and the ability to change.

Change

Remember that yin and yang is about interdependence. Like night and day, one cannot exist without the other.

Successful relationships are therefore about controlling your yin and yang energy as a team to navigate this natural ebb and flow of chi between two people.

How can you do this? Focus on communication and build a strong connection and understanding of your own energy and yin yang states.

5

Support

Together, two people can achieve more than one. To play an equal part in one whole, two complementary forces must mutually support each other.

Think of how yin and yang appear to lean on each other in the Taiji. Both shapes rely on the other to support and hold it.

Flow

Long-lasting relationships will experience huge transformations. Together you may see as much trouble, failure and fatigue, as you will energy, growth and success.

As this belief system suggests, this is the natural rhythm of life and all relationships experience the same circular flow.

Let this truth calm any fears that life is stuck in one place, or that you will not be able to handle the changes coming your way.

"The yin to my yang"

In love, some people believe that meeting your soulmate is like finding your equal opposite.

You may have seen the yin yang symbol used to represent this perfect union of two different people into one blended whole.

This duality is important in relationships, but so is interdependence, dynamism and the sharing of power.

“Yin and yang, male and female, strong and weak, rigid and tender, Heaven and Earth, light and darkness, thunder and lightning, cold and warmth, good and evil… the interplay of opposite principles constitutes the Universe.”

Confucius
(551–479 BCE)

When we balance the yin and yang within us, we make space for true inner peace.

Inner peace

One interpretation of yin yang is that the two opposites never act as peaceful equals. Instead, they are constantly at odds, trying to overcome one another.

By this reasoning, finding peace is not about getting rid of conflict - this is a natural part of life - but it is about learning how to take the rough with the smooth, knowing that change is always around the corner.

Self-reiki for peace

Like acupuncture, reiki is a technique used to improve the flow of energy through the body, but the technique uses gentle touch instead of penetrating the skin - and can be done at home.

Reiki originated in Japan but was heavily inspired by the Chinese notion of balance for an enriched life.

A simplified technique called self-reiki was devised to help unite Heaven (yang) energy, found above, with Earth (yin) energy, found below, at the heart centre by combining basic postures with meditation exercises.

A 5-minute self-reiki practice

- Ground yourself on the floor to connect with Earth and its yin properties.
- Sitting cross-legged, lift your head and straighten your spine to tap into yang energy, above.
- Centre your hands in front of your heart and place your palms together in a prayer position.
- Close your eyes and breathe deeply to help clear your mind.
- Stay here for five minutes without interruption until you feel the energy flowing between your fingertips – uniting yin and yang, above and below.

Meditation

In the western world, stress is one of the most likely factors to throw us off kilter. When work creeps into your personal life, your yang energy of effort and exertion suppresses your yin energy of ease and relaxation at home, leading to an imbalance. Without redressing this equilibrium, stress, anxiety and tension are likely to follow.

Meditation can help. In Chinese culture, this daily discipline is used to "empty" the mind using concentration, mindfulness, contemplation and visualization.

Earth (yin) & Heaven (yang) meditation exercise

When your work-life balance is off, this yin-boosting activity will bring greater harmony to the mind.

- Settle in a restful seated position on the floor with your eyes closed. Stabilize yourself.
- Steady your arms and hands with your fingertips resting on the knees.
- Start your meditation channelling yin: consciousness, presence and awareness.
- Release yang and the busyness of your mind.
- Mentally scan your body. Release any tension in your jaw. Relax your shoulders.
- Stay in this focused yet calm position for five minutes.

Activating Earth energy

Sitting on the floor, feel your tail bone solid and heavy, pressing into the yin of the Earth.

Taking deep breaths, imagine a dark and heavy energy in your lower abdomen (sacral chakra), powerfully rooting you down to the ground.

You are connecting to Earth's yin energy.

Activating Heaven energy

While seated upright or standing, elongate your spine and stretch your neck/head a little taller toward the sky, toward yang.

Draw in vibrant light energy from above through the head (crown chakra). Let it fill your abdomen, illuminating your upper body with energy, air and activity.

You are connecting to Heaven's yang energy.

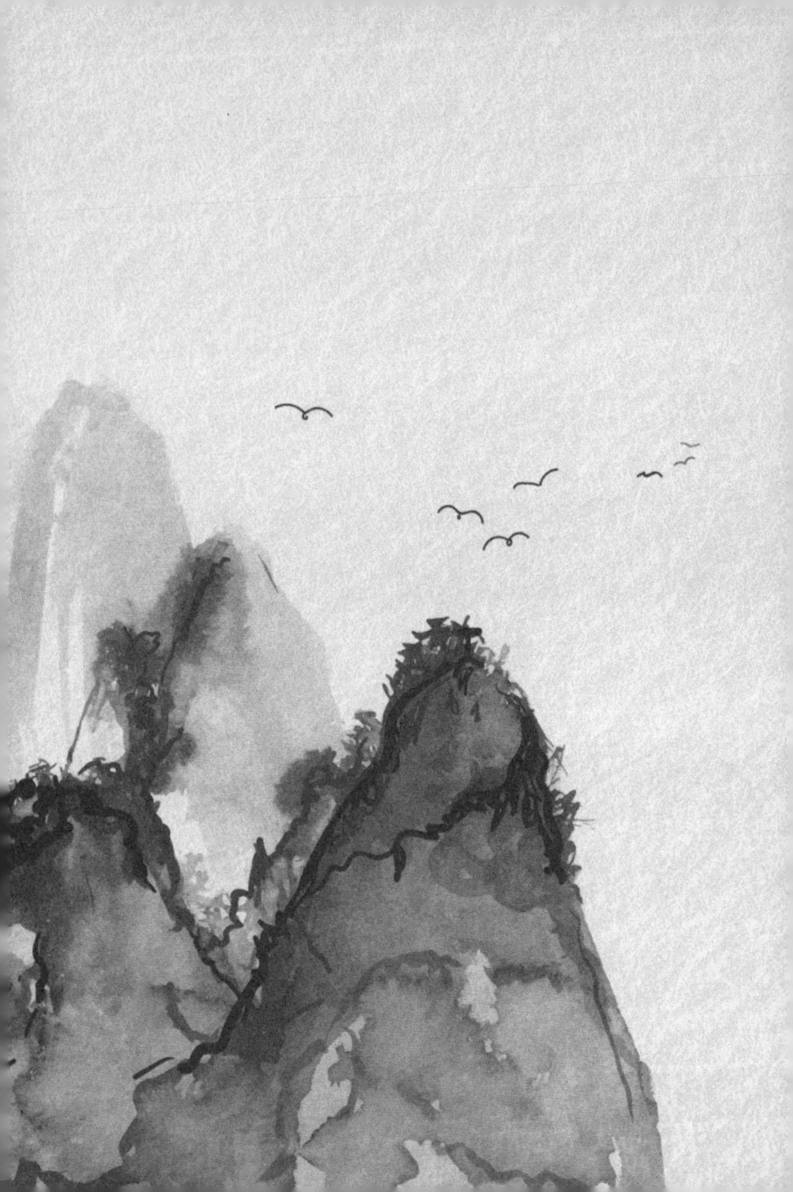

Chapter Four

BALANCE FOR ENVIRONMENT

"You are part of nature and nature is part of you. Do not try to live as if you are separate. You are not. You are part of your family. You are part of your landscape. You are part of the seasons. You are part of both Heaven and Earth."

Martin Palmer,
Yin & Yang, 1997

Harmony starts at home

By now, you might believe that balance is achievable in your health and self, thanks to the principles of yin yang.

In Chinese culture, harmony starts at home and through the pioneering concept of Feng Shui, we can learn how to use yin yang philosophy to create spaces that bring fortune, prosperity and luck.

What is Feng Shui?

Feng Shui encapsulates how we channel the invisible force of chi flowing through us and our environments to live in sync with it.

It is most commonly applied to house layout, but the ancient practice is even used in town planning in China, to decide where classrooms, gyms and offices are built. (Inside them, you'd better believe the boss has the most prosperous seat in the house!)

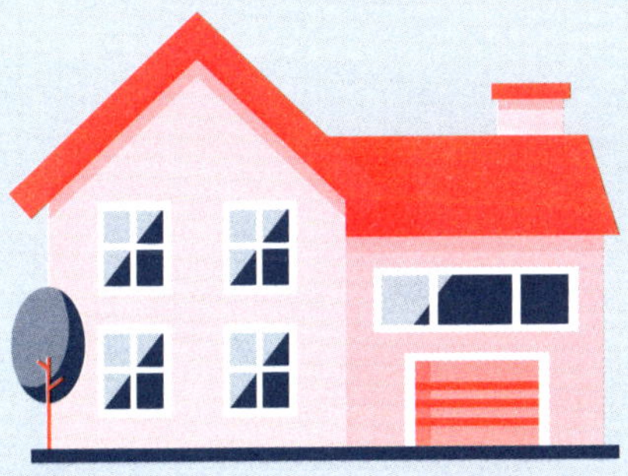

Houses can be designed with Feng Shui concepts at the heart of architectural choices, to make sure chi cannot slip away from the home.

However, it is most commonly seen on a smaller scale, where the art of stabilizing yin and yang is achieved with layout, light, plants and colour palettes.

Interiors

Your home is filled with yin and yang energy. Each room needs its own balance to prevent a feeling of restlessness in predominantly yang spaces or lethargy from excess yin.

There will be family-oriented entertaining areas like the living room and kitchen that naturally boost lively yang energy - but without adding calm accents of yin, rooms can appear crowded, overstimulating or uncomfortable.

Lighting (and the variation of bright and dim) is particularly important for a yin space like the bedroom, where the aim is to create a mood conducive with sleep by night, and wakefulness by morning.

Sources of yin & yang in your home

YIN	**YANG**
Darkness	Light
Cosy corners	Open space
Clutter	Minimalism
Peace & quiet	Loud noises
Cool shades	Bright colours

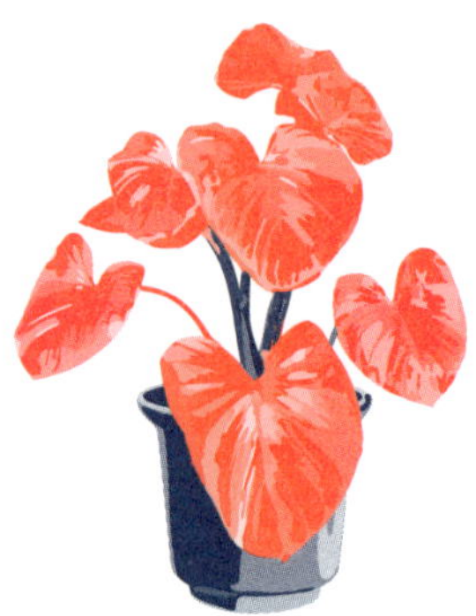

How to arrange your living room

- To maintain a healthy flow of chi, create easy access from the front door to the living room.
- For prosperity, place a leafy green plant underneath the "wealth point", which is believed to be in the top left-hand corner of your living room, as you enter.

How to arrange your bedroom

- ☯ To balance excess yin, position the head of the bed on the east side of the room, as this has the greatest yang energy.
- ☯ For a restful night, avoid positioning the bed behind a door (where intruders are out of sight) or opposite the door (which could drain your chi).

How to arrange your kitchen

- For healthy yin yang balance, keep the oven (yang) away from the fridge (yin), because in nature, the element of fire destroys water.
- Since the kitchen is the heart of the home and a common space for visitors, the cooker should be the focal point because it gives off powerful yang energy.

House hunting with Feng Shui

- Driveways to the side of a house avoid chi fleeing through the front door.
- Money could slip away from homes facing onto a gap between buildings.
- A house dwarfed by larger buildings is at risk of disrupted chi.
- The façade of the building should appear balanced. Think: evenly spaced windows and doors.
- Homes built near a slow-moving stream receive beneficial chi.
- A house built on a triangular plot of land is considered unlucky.

How to arrange your workspace

In a home office, improve your work-life balance by clearly separating your workspace from energetic social areas such as the living room. In a shared office, create a calm sanctuary by applying Feng Shui principles to your desk area.

The optimal desk position would have your chair facing the door (to command control and stability), with a solid, supporting wall behind you. Your computer should be angled away from the glare of a bright window.

Maximize the flow of chi on your desktop by decluttering regularly. Plants inject yang, while a desk water feature promotes soothing yin.

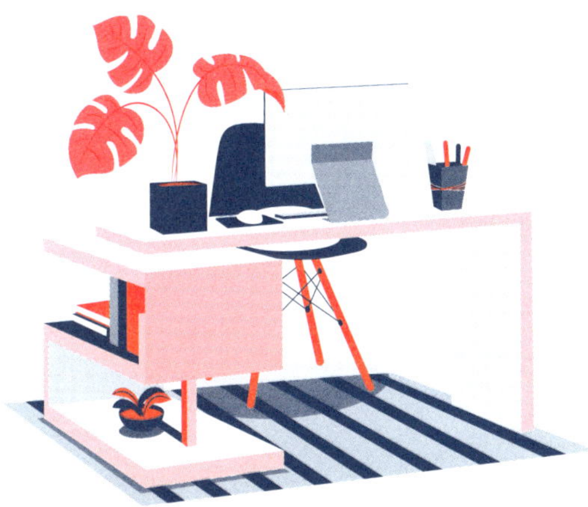

A desk for success

IN	OUT
Plants	Clutter
Organization	Sofa beds
Metal materials	Loud music
Soothing shades (blue, green, purple)	Bright colours (red, orange, yellow)

Yin yang all around

There are many ways that we can control yin and yang energies in our home and work environments, but living in harmony with the natural elements goes back to the roots of this ancient philosophy.

Ultimately, we are all living at the mercy of the energy that ebbs and flows around us and although we can find areas to control, for the most part we must learn how to let nature take its course.

Daoists advocate "active inaction", meaning we must tune into the order of the Universe while effectively moving with it and "going with the flow" to avoid violence, suffering and struggle.

How to tune into the elements

Experience wild swimming

Exercise outside regularly

Take a walk after an evening meal

Feel the earth beneath bare feet

Eat in the great outdoors

Step outside when it's raining

Feel the sunshine on your skin

Gaze at the Moon at night

Watch a flame as it flickers

The Dao way of life

Can you tell your yin from your yang?

Hopefully you have learned that life is not black and white – you cannot have yin without yang, and vice versa.

As the Taiji symbol represents, yin and yang are in continuous flow. This is the Dao way of life and it reflects the constant interplay between ever-changing yin and yang.

“Yin and Yang are one vital force – the primordial aura.”

Wang Yang-Ming,
The Philosophy of Wang Yang-Ming, 1916

The secret of yin yang is *you*

Instead of trying to resist adversity or fight our differences, you must lean into them and understand that change is inevitable.

Accept every part of yourself. Tune into your energy, and be aware of your emotions and what you might need.

Go with the flow. Adapt, change, grow and prosper.

“The heart of a human being is no different from the soul of Heaven and Earth. In your practice always keep in your thoughts the interaction of Heaven and Earth, water and fire, yin and yang.”

Morihei Ueshiba,
The Art of Peace, 1991